THE WAY
BACK

Poems of Addiction & Recovery

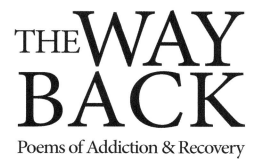

THE WAY BACK

Poems of Addiction & Recovery

Michael Landfair

Huertas Press

Huertas #9

San Miguel de Allende, GTO, Mexico 37700

San Miguel de Allende 2017

ISBN: 978-0-9990091-0-9

From The Big Book: Me An Alcoholic?

Barleycorn's wringer squeezed this author--but he escaped quite whole.

The Birthday Coin

I squeeze your birthday coin in my palm
celebrating your years of sobriety
stamped in Roman numerals on its face.
Flat and cold, the number reveals nothing
about the depths you reached.

One ex-drunk after another
around the room encloses
the coin in a fist to record
the best arguments against
taking that first drink for the next year.

My coin is my constant companion.
Sometimes, when I want a drink
I run my finger across the raised number
as if it were a scar.

A Trial By Questions

DWF called saying her name was Marina.
She roused me from a nap, recharging
from the stress of too many early mornings,
hot stocks, meetings without point.

She had the money voice; that teeth-together
Bryn Mahr way of speaking. When she spoke,
I heard opera, Arabian horses and Wimbledon.
It was tight like a good jazz trio.
Not filled with the awkward and redundant
you knows of the young.

What are your interests? Where have you traveled?
She compelled and challenged me to work harder.
The way it must be to play Jimmy Connors.
But, I was rusty and loose
used to easy banter with clients and friends.

The old insecurities of being Eastside,
my parents' eastside, blue collar workers,
middle-class values, and nightmares of moving back,
came whispering. I struggled, failed to move my feet,
tossed defensive lobs, and Connors said with a smirk
Nice game.

Robin's Sculpture

For fifty years through changing seasons
the walnut tree stood in her front yard
recording in its cells the life of Onyx Street.

And stored inside,
was the love of Robin's parents
the night they conceived her:

The sound of her cries for attention, the sibling rivalry,
the alcoholic ranting of the neighbors next door,
and her first boyfriend, who flaunted authority,

with his leather jacket, and cigarette smoke
and English Leather
and her palpitating heart

caused by his kisses;
the pain in the carved heart
Dean loves Robin on its trunk.
the U of O marching band

with its clarinets and horns and the beat
to the music that was stored within.

And stored, too, were the distant cheers
from the stadium as Bobby Moore
gathered in another pass and scored a touchdown;

the peace marches
and the *Hell no we won't go*
and the love-ins

and the Beatles, in those cells.
The branches cradled the telephone lines
that vibrated with love and laughter

sorrow and anger,
sometimes in foreign tongues.
The recordings of love on Onyx stopped on
Columbus Day,

when mighty winds from the south pulled its roots
from the ground.
And in that stacked pile of memories at the curb

was a log whose grain held the life of the street.

An artist carved that piece of walnut into a sculpture of a girl.

If you take a long look

I swear, you might see movement in the grain.

Hear the voices

Experience the history, as she did.

You might even faintly smell the English Leather

if you weren't distracted by the clarinets.

Dead Horse Point, Utah

At Dead Horse Point, great canyons stretch before me.

The setting sun backlights the scudding clouds.

A gentle breeze, loaded with the smell of Junipers, whispers

of the desert to the south. The shawl of evening cloaks

the sandstone boulders.

Under the stars of Orion a red fox yips in the dying light.

I traveled much of a lifetime to this place to see a sunset.

Moving Day

I travel light
> when I move in with a lady
> I don't disturb her décor.
> only problem...you can't tell I live there.

I am a new male Model American
> my ex-wives are housekeepers.
> What I own fits in your standard four-door sedan.

It's moving day back to the same apartment complex
> with the same floor plan...
> I know from experience
> where to put my hairdryer.

Tennis with My Daughter

What BETTER   way   to SPEND

               the day

Than HITTING   to   my DAUGHTER

We NEVER   played   This GAME

The WAY   we really   OUGHT to.

YELLS   and   SCREAMS

           And

COACHES   WORDS

were no

SUBSTITUTE   for   FUN.

Three YEARS   have changed   the COACH

              I see

To a FRIEND   when the   GAME

              is DONE.

Tausha

Have a nice life! she said

punctuated by my car door.
She marched away
head high.

Then she turned
her demeanor thawed and said
You know I always loved you
I count you among my friends
I was willing to try again,
but I see you've changed your mind
I really wish you well...
it hurts to see you drive away

Two years before
roles reversed
she stood at our door
and watched me pack my car
I inched away to mother's house

watched for some sign,
some small tic
of a mistake.

It hurt so much to go.

The Dream

It startled me awake, the dream
of a sewer in the basement
snaking off to terror.

My shadow ran to catch and passed me
as I scuttled before the rats and brushed
spiders from my back.

I emerged into a lighted room
and paused to rest,
but shrank before another mouth of doom.

Like movie stars on movie screens
who go to basements in the dark
I could not resist. I had to see what's there.

It's a secret or a sickness
about that thing that lurks
out of sight and in the mind

in some bowel-deep pool where my adult anger
brews
of rabbit ears and kittens dropped down wells,
on that farm that smelled of poplars, when I was six.

The Vietnam Memorial 1991

I walked that circular path to 1968–1969.
With my arms around me,
barely holding on.
In white letters between *Lonnie D. Moore and Gary
B. Hogson,*
my fraternity brother, *Max F. DeSully, Jr.*

I sat and stared through tears
at the black mirrored surface
scarred with death.

A couple walked up and reflected color
through the pain:
they stopped in front of *Edward L. Handy.*
He's from Salem, she said.
He wouldn't back down from anybody, said he.
Do you have someone here?

With their dad, two boys 13 and 11 gaped
at the dead boys' names.

The couple walked up together, hand in hand.
He stood silently and stiffly as he captured the name
from the wall, then walked off alone.

Terry L. Thompson
I went to school with him, he said.
He squatted and ran his fingers across his name,
quiet as if in silent prayer.
When at last he walked away, he stopped and
briefly looked back.

I sat alone and saw my reflection amidst the names.
The tears came no more.
I said goodbye to Max for now.

Alone

Alone is that storm in winter light
that pushes dry snow before the wind
and I sit before the fireplace close
snugged away for safety.

I am familiar with being alone.
Alone is putting up shutters
shutting down so as not to feel pain
steeling myself from it happening again.

Depression

Boy, I think I'm in trouble here
I'm going down the drain.

This pit's a maelstrom
where my navel used to be.

My feet, my hands, my head
are all that's left of me.

Help me God, I howled.
My head spins past my feet,

I can't remember when things weren't sad
and I can't will the gloom to lift.

and that black hole
blots out the brightest day
with its ebon shawl of grief.

Two years, 17 days ago today

It was exactly 2 years, 17 days ago today.

I remember where I was
I stood on the corner of Oak Street
and hollered out her name.

You're the one who made me hate you
you're the one I blame
I can feel it painful now
as it was just then.

It was 10:15 in the morning
I was sucking on a straw
filling my head with poison
don't want to live just now.

It was 2 years 17 days ago today.

I remember exactly where I was
I was on the corner of Oak street
talking about my loss
you're the one who made me love you.

You'll always be the same.

I soaked my heart in alcohol
and anesthetized my brain
it was 2:00 in the morning
won't you please go home?

I'll call you, if I have your number
did you get all your clothes?
It was exactly 2 years 17 days ago today
I stood in the shadow of an oak tree.

I remember exactly where I was.

Sonny

He hadn't seen his mom in years
and much was left unfinished.
He called home and when she answered, he said
Hi mama, this is sonny.
Sonny who?
Your son, mama.

She hung up and that stab went through him
and I felt it, too
I shrank in my chair
and stared at the ceiling while others related stories
about their mamas and papas.

The worst thing that could happen wasn't death.
It was watching someone you cared about suffer.
We were like tornados in our family's lives
expecting to be forgiven when the storm was over.

Beverly

Peek-a-Boo

The boy in me remembers...
I peeked from behind her full skirt
and laughed
when I was caught looking
and ducked back behind again.
It was peek-a-boo.
A game all children played.

This time I'm an adult.
That feeling of playing that game
was present.
I quickly stared
trying to take in as much as possible
in short bursts of staring
at this woman with her expressive eyes
her artistic poses
her face that changed expressions
like a diamond reflecting the light.

When I was caught peeking
embarrassed that she could mean
so much to me
in such a short time

I laughed.

Homage to Other Poets

Work
A Tribute to N Scott Momaday

I

Robins wing at dawn to worms. Raccoons
sift the shallows for crawdads. Je t'aime,
she sighs as squirrels swoop to walnut trees,
and I leave my home for work.

II

Under fluorescents, phones ring
in unseen places. Voices, perhaps
recorded by the long departed, spew words
as screens track fortunes made and lost.

III

Grandpa lifts his John Deere hat and soaks-up
sweat with his sleeve. Grandma calls "come boss"
to the Guernseys. Straight shadowed furrows stitch
the warm earth and he makes his way to the barn.

Blue Red White

Bright big boy
in a blue baby bed
sings the blues
and sobs for the dead.

Red Robin roosting
in the Russian rains
reads Dostoevsky
as he writhes in his chains.

When winter whips
where wonder was to be
a wafer thin whistle
wails for you and me.

Tribute to Billy Collins: Directions

You Know the Via del Renatti?

You know the Via del Renatti
the street you find on the south side of Via del Corso
the street that runs parallel to the Tavare River
where the Italian bookstore is?
And you know how if you leave the street
and walk into the narrow alley you come
to the Trattoria Grigio in an ocher
building from the 1500's
an oasis of tables and chairs
fenced by the green boxwood
amid the buzzing of Vespa's?
And farther on, you know
the columned cathedral with
the brick-lined moat
and if you go beyond that you arrive
at the Piazza Navarno?
Well, if you start walking and you
might have to dodge and say "scuzie"
when it's crowded with tourists
you will come to the Pantheon
a large stone edifice with Corinthian columns
and a good place to stop.

The best time is late afternoon
when the sun casts shadows
on the Medieval buildings circling the square
wrought iron balconies draped in Solumna,
white and pink flowers catching the light.
And when you find an agreeable
place to sit on the inside
there the hole in the dome
provides the only source of light
you will be able to see the tomb of Raphael
and the Imperial Marble on the floor
and in a broad band around the room.

And if this is your day,
you might even hear from 2000 years away
the praise and prayer to the
Roman gods.

My Father

My Father, His Son

My father was raised by a railroad man.
There wasn't much money in Steerman.
A quarter would buy a bucket of milk, a loaf of bread
and a penny candy.
Dad taught me the Lord's Prayer and the 23rd Psalm
at my bedside.
I lived for his approval. I watched for some sign that
he loved me.

The news each morning was served by a slow waiter.
My father and I would sit at the kitchen counter and
argue for hours.
We fought over Vietnam. I yelled that it was a civil
war.
He said we were there to save the people. He called
me a damned
Communist. Me, who scratched "I Love Barry Gold-
water" in the sand!

I'll be fifty-seven next January. That 24-year-old in
the mirror
just escapes my eyes. The news seems disposable,
not worth an effort,
like that trout that just noses the fly on a hot summer
day.

That black wall
in DC haunts me. We could have won, but for the
politicians, and today,
Max De Sully would be alive,
not shot by a sniper weeks after his honeymoon.

Dad now thinks we had no business being in Viet
Nam.
It was a quagmire.
Our government was wrong; we had no national
interests to defend.
I am sick of the massive government in our lives.
Dad now fears
for his Medicare and Social Security. He votes for all
the liberals.
My father and I have a skittishness about us.
My father is now the Communist.

I Dreamt of Sgt. Kowasch

I had heard so many stories about army life. I feared
what was coming and yet my father said, *The army
will make a man out of you.* I feared Viet Nam more
I just knew that terrible things awaited me over there,
if
I didn't avoid the draft. My other choice was Canada,
never to see my friends and family again.

Sgt Kowasch remembered our company,
made up of mostly reservists.
He remembered how we had excelled at training and
remembered
how hard he made it on us for avoiding combat. We
talked
for awhile about those times, while he drank his beer.

One thing I shared with Kowasch was
how the army helped me.
I found when things got tough in life,
as they do for most of us,
I could look back on my experiences and have confi-
dence
that this too, I could get through.

As we reminisced, a slightly overweight and soft
looking kid
hung on our conversation.
If war broke out tomorrow with China, he interjected,
What should I do?
I remembered my father's words to his anxious son,
which seem more true today:
Go into the army, I said, *The army will make a man
out of you.*

Valerie

The Roosters didn't wake her
80 years a wife and mother, my aunt
my father's sister.

Valerie, we love you.

We gathered in the chapel
wrapped in arms to view her, the brother
and the brother's son
and nieces, daughters of the one
who didn't waken.

Valerie, can you hear me?

And in the chapel
memories crept on carpet feet.
And all who loved her, mourned her
for our remaining time upon this earth.

Valerie, can you hear me?

Observations of a Poet

Code words

They're on the airwaves
they're in the news
words that you and I couldn't use
when we were kids.

You douche bag!

Douche bags and condoms
used on places we didn't know we had
when we were kids.

No body function's sacred.
Ad agencies bill time in millions.

Sexual Reassignment
Nutrient Dense
Monostat 7
Femcare
Immodium–ID
Gynelotrium

Mort Sahl and Lenny Bruce
knew all the words
that were scandalous to say aloud.
And now those words are flaunted
before daughters, on the silver screens.

My First Track Meet

Too small for football and no interest in team sports,
my event was the first leg of a 660 relay.
I had trained in tennis shoes and sweats weighted
for weeks by the rain.

There I stood in lane eight, last event
of the day. (My parents said they would try
to make it. I anxiously scanned the faces
of the crowd.)

My feet March cold numbed
in thin-soled spikes crunched the volcanic rock.
Like a deer breaking cover
I started fast in those shoes and gathered
in the distance.

I was leading after one lap.

I gasped past the starting line
heard my coaches and teammates yell
Cut for the Pole!
Cut for the Pole!

I should have known what that meant.
On legs like a baby just starting to walk,
my lungs on fire, I passed on the baton
in my outside lane,

that night over dinner, my parents asked,
How did you do?
I finished second!

I Didn't Know Katharine Hepburn

I did not know Katharine Hepburn,
but name her movies and I'm back in the Aladdin
Theater,
my popcorn topped with real butter, as Katherine
worries words like a dog's toy.

I did not know Elvis Presley,
but play "Blue Moon", and I am at the Father-Daugh-
ter banquet
wishing I had black curly hair and a sneer on my lip,
as my band sings that song.

I knew Evelyn Dickson,
my sixth-grade teacher who gave me *Outlaw of the
Sorrel Land*
the year I was in an oxygen tent. She taught me to
love words.
I wish I could hear her voice.

I know Amber who cannot speak to me
other than in barks.
I just want to hear she loves me in any kind of voice.

How Will We Remember This Day?

Light prisms flicker off the crystal tipped
to the oenophiles' nose. Mozart's Requiem
weaves through the conversations. Cashmere
drapes
from tanned and powdered shoulders.

The providers of orthodontists' vacations
with their Cole Haan tassels and tinted hair,
used to the smell of Polo and Poison,
cannot smell the breath of war.

Mud-caked boots foul the hardwood floors.
Its stink of wars wafts from its body.
Two eyes like sewers catch the glint
of light from the glasses and gold necklaces.

Like a mirror, those eyes reflect pictures,
you can see them if you look,
of grandfathers and young boys weeping
for fallen warriors.

Killed A Bug

I killed a bug the other day for fun
squashed between the sink and tub.
Not one second passed
life snuffed out, but here's the rub

Is it that easy to take a life?
Or is the difference the size?
Could a large husband take out a small wife
or think a moment, otherwise?

Our World

The world keeps spinning faster
like that steel merry-go-round
filled with my playmates,
on my playground.
Pushed faster and faster
by the neighborhood bullies
today's clowns of madness
until we're horizontal,
barely holding on.
Pushing faster
slippery fingers
flying missiles
But I just learned Patience!!
And the clowns are convulsed with laughter.

Little Jimmy

Little Jimmy had a shoeshine stand
on the corner of Fifth and Pine.
Men would sit and watch
him whip his rag
with a pop! And a pop, pop, pop!
a beat in double time.
Johnny wanted to be like Jimmy.
He labored day and night
to slather polish in black and brown
so his shoes would reflect the light.
But no one could beat little Jimmy
he had a secret sauce
one part spit & polish
the rest was the way he'd toss
his hair from side to side
and ride the rag in double time
to the end of the watcher's line.

Under Red Washed Skies

Under red washed skies, the couple came to dine.
She sat forward and like a magician,
pulled topics from around his ears.

Silently upright in his straight-backed chair,
he shifted his gaze, avoided her eyes.

She prodded him with words like spears
he fumbled for a pocketed cigarette
and brushed at her words
as if they were flies.

Collapsing back, a sigh escaped the woman's lips.

He reached with upturned palm
To cup her graying hair.

I'd like to think
I'd like to think
He saw the girl
no longer there.

Morning In Woodstock

Last night white-tailed deer,
all pivot and dash,
high-stepped like drum majorettes
down the fence line
in the knee-deep snow.

Black shocks of birch and ash,
solemn skeletons, keep lookout,
as sumac, like sergeants, shush with
red brush hands, and crimson mists
of salmon berries hang in the air.

Platoons of firs, planted
since the fire,
branches bound in snow like cotton,
stand in long lines at attention.

In my robe, coffee cold,
I search far into the woods
from the window,
for some movement
some stir of wind.

The Garden

There is a little garden
high up in the woods
where froggies croak
and old women hang clothes of fire
on lines meant for peapods.

Ash Wednesday

Ash Wednesday is a fine day to travel.
The Ford, plump with boxes of worn-outs
filled to the wooden side rails, waits
for Ma, the kids and me.

This fertile land drew us like Magi. It now
lays broken, fine as flour, under the windows.
Dirt, so dry it will wring the promises,
rubs our houses sore.

The Sheridan Hotel scoured clean
by the wind that cowboys ride
on the theater marquee. Names of stars lean
like tombstones on Boot Hill.

The kerchiefs of wailing women, flap on poles
dusky waves of cottonwoods line wheel
ruts that crash like dreams on outcrops
sharp as broken bones.

THE RIVER

We walked through the open door
down to the river.

DOWN TO THE RIVER

We filled our blank page
with the sounds of children
who curl like a snake.

CURLS LIKE A SNAKE

Back and forth under the gentle sun
through the art in the plaza.
Life is not meant just
for the fountain of youth,
but for you and me.

FOR YOU AND ME

Let the music in the sky
overwhelm our field of vision.

LET THE MUSIC IN THE SKY
OVERWHELM OUR FIELD OF
VISION.

Wind, Wave, Artichoke, Listen, Thunder

Listen to the wind
shaking the chime in the key of D.

Wave after wave of rushing air
slices through the pepper tree
upsetting the nest of grackles.

Listen to the thunder announce
the coming rain
washing the fields of artichokes..

Smell the rain coax
the dust from the earth.

Acknowledgements

I want to acknowledge the gifts I've received from teachers who cared about what I wrote.

There's Doug Marx in Portland, part of Willamette Writers who hyped me up on poets and filled my brain with creativity.

The writers group here in San Miguel consisting of Florence Grande, Lynda Schor, John Scherber, Christina Johnson, Marcia Loy, and Dr. Cynthia Miller. They gave me a safe place to fail and learn and inspired me with their use of language.

There's Chet Kozlowski who gave me all sorts of encouragement writing a novel.

And not least, the effervescent Judyth Hill. Everytime I turn around I think of some story or snippet of poem read aloud by her that inspires me.

Finally, My wife Beverly. She continued to support me and encouraged me to do better.

One last thing...

When you move to the next page, Kindle will give you the opportunity to rate this collection of poems and share your thoughts through an automatic feed to your Facebook and Twitter accounts. If you enjoyed The Way Back and think others will too, your input will be greatly appreciated.

Please consider posting a review on Amazon to recommend this book to other poetry lovers.

To get a free copy of the next book from Michael Landfair plus my monthly newsletter, please email me at landfair3554@gmail.com. Once you confirm your email, you'll receive your book and email.

Thank you and happy reading.

All the best, Michael